Thyroid First Aid Kit
'A 3-step guide to healing the thyroid.'

Stephanie Powers
2017

Thyroid First Aid Kit

Copyright © 2017 by STEPHANIE POWERS

ISBN-13: 978-1979604215
ISBN-10: 1979604215

Printed in the United States of America

Dedication

To my mother Lisa who courageously carried me in her womb while simultaneously battling thyroid cancer.

Look at the ripple effect you have created.

I love you.

Acknowledgements

Special thanks to Rebecca Hinson at Rebecca Hinson Art (https://www.rebeccahinson.com) for bringing my vision of the cover to life beyond my expectations. I am eternally grateful for our instant bond over vegan smoothies that one day in May!

Thank you Kylie Connolly for being the first set of eyes on this book to make sure it was in tip-top shape before being released. Your editing skills are unmatched. The Universe conspired to bring us together... of that I'm sure.

Thank you to my husband Mitch for pushing me to make my dream of being an author a reality; For always making sacrifices to support my dreams. Thank you for allowing me to write so openly about our relationship. You are one of a kind Mitch — I'll never find another like you. I love you always.

A huge thank you to my mother Lisa who allowed me to rest at her home in New Hampshire so I could focus on pouring my energy into this book. Thank you, mama, for opening up and bravely sharing every detail of your story so that I could in turn share it with the world. Remember all the times we would come up with clever phrases and shout... 'Book Title!'

Look. I actually did it.

To all of the people who pre-ordered this book, you were the fan to my flame during the entire process. I appreciate you all SO incredibly much for your support. Words cannot express.

Finally, to all of the people this book mentions either by description or by name... thank you for molding me into the person I am today. Without your pain, love, disappointment, or joy, I would not be a published author today. Gratitude.

Thyroid
First Aid Kit

'A 3-step guide
to healing the thyroid.'

Stephanie Powers
2017

Contents

Foreword

Hi. My name is Stephanie Powers. I'm the voice behind the words of Thyroid First Aid Kit, and the daughter of a woman who survived thyroid cancer.

I never wanted to be known as the 'thyroid girl' or even become a holistic health coach. To be honest, I never really gave much thought about my health until my diagnosis. As a child, I grew up eating mac'n'cheese and washing it down with Kool-aid. In college, I drank more red bulls than any human should and my diet consisted of salads covered in cheese and ranch dressing. *Yup. That girl is now writing a health book.*

I graduated from Southern New Hampshire University in 2011 with a degree in Organizational Leadership and no idea what I wanted to do with it. I wound up at an entry level job at a health insurance company where the next few years of my life were routine and bland. Well… during work anyway. At home, they were chaotic and traumatic.

On March 31st 2011, I was woken up by what sounded like someone violently breaking into the house. I jumped out of bed faster than I ever have before and ran downstairs; my fight or flight senses ready to flip a car. I turn the corner after the last step and my eyes dialate in spine tingling shock as I find my brother face up on the ground next to a flipped over kitchen table, a face as dark as midnight, eyes rolled back white, and foam pouring out of his mouth. He was having a severe grand mal seizure on the kitchen floor. I ran over to him and began screaming his name. Not having a clue on how to save him, I start scooping foam out of his mouth (never do this) as tears began to drop on his blue face. The sound of his heavy limbs banging on the hard wood floor as I cried to the 911 operator that my brother was dying, is a noise etched into my memory forever.

He was diagnosed with epilepsy a few months and a few more seizures later. Watching a grand mal seizure is still, to this day, one of the most traumatic experiences of my life. The way my mom checks his pulse and looks up at me with nervous eyes as she cant feel anything. The bloody head wounds from falling, the two black eyes from lack of oxygen.. it never get's easier seeing your brother like that.

Six months after this traumatic night, I became engaged, and in June 2013 I eloped on a beach in Key West after an extremely emotional period of wedding planning. My new husband and I promptly moved a thousand miles away from home after we returned from our honeymoon. I quit my job at the health insurance company and ran away to South Carolina looking for a fresh start where no one knew my name.; I desperately wanted to escape life in New Hampshire. The dead end job, the awful memories from school, and thte trauma from my brothers new disease. Life in South Carolina was starting to feel free and fun, but then something happened.

Six months after we moved, at a routine OBGYN appointment, I was diagnosed with an autoimmune disease called Hashimotos Thyroiditis. I know what you're thinking --- "Hashi-what?" I thought that too. Getting diagnosed with an autoimmune disease that Western medicine deems 'incurable' was one of the scariest moments of my life. Being told my chances of ever having a baby are slim to none is the *last* thing a newly-wed wants to hear.

———◆———

Do you believe in the mantra 'everything happens for a reason'? I sure do. I've become so good at trusting this, that even when trauma strikes, I ride the wave and trust that I'll soon see why this had to happen. Looking back at my diagnosis in 2014, and all the events leading up to it, I'm really glad it all happened. It was the Universe placing 'orange cones' on my path to keep me in line with my destiny of becoming a holistic health professional. If I were never diagnosed, there would be countless women laying under the knife in an operating room about to get their thyroid removed. If I were never exposed to trauma, I couldn't connect on a deep level with my clients suffering from anxiety. If I were never diagnosed with an autoimmune disease, this book would not be in your hands…

The book you're holding may seem like any other book. But what lies in your hands is a collection of healing energy that I absorbed while on many hikes — by myself — in the woods of South Carolina. My hyperthyroid made my anxiety intense, so when I discovered that the cure for racing thoughts was right outside my window, I became addicted to being in the woods. I hiked in the snow, in blistering heat, through a thunderstorm — I even went out during Hurricane Matthew. Every single day I met 'myself' in the woods to take a long, therapeutic walk. The pine trees were my therapist as I held conversations out loud, the wind confirmed my premonitions, and any negative voices telling me 'you can't do this' were washed away by the rivers I crossed. What you hold in your hands was created by synchronistic encounters in the deserts of Colorado, and sudden epiphanies that developed deep in the jungles of Florida. What you hold in your hands, should you choose to follow each instruction carefully, has the power to completely change your life.

Close the book and flip through the pages — like a deck of cards. The same force creating wind in your face is what pushed me to create this for you. I came up with the 'First Aid Kit' concept because when I was diagnosed with Hashimotos, I didn't care about anything besides how I could heal it — and quick, because I just wanted to get back to my normal life of being a newlywed in a new city. I just wanted the basics without a detailed discussion on TSH, T3, T4 and the pituitary gland.

———◆———

So there I was. Twenty-five years old, supposedly in the prime of my health, growing ridges on my fingernails and losing my beautiful hair in chunks. My face was swollen and I was suffering from bloating so bad I looked 7 months pregnant. I had the worst afternoon fatigue and allergies so severe that I bought tissues in bulk every month. I was lonely, because I just moved to a new city and trying to make new friends while battling thyroid-induced anxiety is no easy task. I went through waves of depression so intense that I felt nothing at all; numb. So utterly disconnected from myself and my soul. When I couldn't look at my pets and feel the same love that I used to, or when music became more of an annoyance than joy, I knew something was wrong.

I hid this side of me from everyone because I never

wanted to be a burden. (You'll see in Chapter 3 why this played a huge role in harming my thyroid.) At 25, I should have been out socializing with other 20-somethings, or building a career in something I loved. But I was too tired, physically and mentally, to do any of that. Instead I spent all of my free time alone reading thick 300+ page books on the thyroid and it's role in the body.

I sacrificed a few years of my twenties because I refused to accept my diagnosis of being reliant on a pill for LIFE. I was already a slave to student loans, I was not about to become a slave to big pharma.

In December of 2016, I was staying at an airbnb out in Big Pine Key, FL celebrating my 28th birthday. I was laying in a hammock late one night watching the stars, listening to the heavy palm trees blow in the wind. I closed my eyes to rock in the hammock while the echo of the neighbor's seashell wind chime started to jingle when it hit me — I need to quit my job at the health insurance company. I need to do it. I have no idea how I'll pay my rent or my car or my health insurance, but that doesn't matter anymore. There is no more time to waste.

I opened my eyes and saw a shooting star, then my phone lit up with 11:11. So I went home and did it. 'Wow, are you sure?' is the response I kept receiving. My intuition was so strong that not one person's skepticism swayed my mind. While at times I was left shaking in my boots, trying to remain confident that I made the right decision, the Universe would always send me daily notes of reassurance that I was following the right path. These signs mostly came through numbers like 11:11, 2:22, 3:33, etc. but again, that is a whole other story to be published in a future book. Throughout this whole journey, from an initial thought to the hard copy of this book in your hands, the Universe kept telling me:

> *"Do not dig up in fear what you planted in faith."*

Since I took the leap of faith to work for myself, I have devoted my time working 1:1 with courageous women battling thyroid issues. I have helped them get rid of anxiety, grow their hair back, conceive a child, and I've even helped some women dodge major surgery.

It's through my own research, education, and experiences working with clients that has led me to summarize the top three things people have done to successfully bring the thyroid back into balance. Some have even shrunk nodules! It's important to keep in mind that this is a very condensed version of what it takes to heal — so if you find one of the three topics in Thyroid First Aid Kit strikes you as something that may be causing your thyroid issue, do further research. Also important to keep in mind is that everyone is bio-individual. This book will work miracles for some, but show little to no progress for others. This is your soul journey. You know your body better than anyone else…

It is not normal that it has become normal for someone to say they have a thyroid issue. I was terrified at how many women responded with a resounding 'ME TOO!' when I began sharing my diagnosis. I'll never forget the day I was sitting in a Starbucks in Mount Pleasant, South Carolina when I decided to Google the most prescribed pills in America, pondering if thyroid was on the list. To my surprise, not only was it on the most prescribed list but it was #1 for five years running. Holy shit! Why isn't this on CNN? Why isn't this headline news on my Facebook page? My adrenaline took over as I yelled across the coffee shop to share this news with my husband standing in line for coffee, who's only response was a confused glance. "Why isn't everyone freaking out with me?!" I anxiously thought. Relying on a daily pill to live a normal life is anything but normal. My adrenaline calmed into courage, and I instantly became determined to figure out this epidemic. Everyone deserves to live a life free from depression, fatigue, and excess weight. No one should live with panic attacks, heart palpitations, and insomnia. No one should ever unnecessarily have one of their most vital organs removed from their body.

So please... Read this book carefully, then hand it down to anyone you know suffering from a thyroid condition. And when your doctor tells you that your dysfunctional thyroid is genetic, tell them this:

> *"Genes load the gun. Lifestyle pulls the trigger."*

What follows next is the powerful story of how my mother miraculously grew my life while simultaneously growing the thyroid cancer that was trying to take both her life and mine. This is followed by my personal story with Hashimotos, and finally, the Thyroid First Aid Kit - three steps to bring your thyroid back into balance.

Introduction

I'm not supposed to be here.

It's 1988 and I'm just a helpless fetus in the womb. My whole life depends on this beautiful, 28-year-old woman with long, pin straight brown hair and forest green eyes. This vessel I call mother spends her days working the line at a plastics factory in Southern Indiana. I'm stretching her belly out by the day, making it a burden in the way of trimming all the freshly melted plastic that spews out of a machine next to us. Mother likes to ask for breaks to go outside for a breath of fresh air for us, but typically gets denied this luxury.

Her coworkers aren't the nicest people either; the most empathy they've ever expressed has been pointing out a red lump on her neck. She was too exhausted to ever worry about it, though, as she figured it was just another pregnancy symptom. Mother is so beautiful on the outside…it's rare a set of eyes isn't on her. But inside, her heart and mind are suffering greatly. She is always pouring from an empty cup.

In between her mindless duties on the factory line, her thoughts bounce between anger, sadness, and frustration. All she dreams of is a happy, healthy family and a career she can be proud of; none of which are going as planned. She questions the point of life, and why she's wasting so much time working a job she hates. It pays the bills and makes her dad proud, so she carries on, marking her fifth year there. At first, she blames these all-encompassing negative thoughts on the baby blues - she just gave birth to a little boy less than a year ago and her only resource for help is a book from the library. But as she rubs her round, 7-month pregnant belly, she begins to notice that depression isn't her only symptom. She's so exhausted all the time that she can barely lift her arms to rub her own belly. Her long hair, draped all the way down her back, is severely thinning. Her once healthy nails are now brittle.

One day, she wakes up for work unable to get out of bed. Her muscles are so weakened that it takes every ounce of strength just to pull the covers off. With her 1-year-old son screaming and a husband never around to help, she decides she can no longer work at the factory; a hard conclusion for such a hard worker to come to. At this point, she knows something is physically wrong and she's determined to figure out what. With a hint of optimism but mostly defeat, she takes a deep breath as she squints her eyes in pain and rolls out of bed. She makes it to the phone to call the plastics factory to resign. After this, she immediately phones the doctor.

She arrives at the doctor's office that same day. In a cold, windowless room she sits on the exam table as crunchy paper crinkles beneath her. She is shivering; but that's nothing new — being cold all the time has just become a part of who she is. The doctor walks in and begins taking her vitals. As she takes deep breaths in between the doctor moving his cold stethoscope around her chest, he stops to lift his brow and take a step back. Without saying a word he reaches for a hand mirror. He holds it out in front of her, revealing a pale, tired face with the life gone from her eyes.

"Do you see that?" said the doctor.

"No?" my mother said in a tired tone. She was too distracted by how sickly she looked and the sad realization that she hadn't looked in a mirror in weeks.

She held the mirror and watched as the doctor gently palpated her neck and explained, "This is your thyroid. A normal thyroid has a small, butterfly-like shape. Do you see this red lump?" He gently squeezed the delicate skin on her neck to reveal a hard, golf ball size lump on her throat.

"This is not normal. We need to perform a biopsy immediately to see if this is cancer."

My mom squinted her eyes in confusion. Cancer wasn't a word she was familiar with; none of her friends or family ever had that health issue. She felt more confused than fearful as she made her way to the front desk to schedule her biopsy. Just as this new, challenging chapter in life was beginning, she was already praying for the day it would be over.

It was two weeks later when my mother returned to the same windowless exam room. The same doctor inserted a long needle into the golf ball size lump in her throat, but failed to find any results. After nearly an hour of picking and prodding, they both agreed she would need to schedule a second biopsy with a specialist.

It was a week later when my mother meets with an Endocrinologist. She feels frustrated that nobody can figure out what is wrong with her. With what little energy she has left from this mysterious disease, she hates that she has to spend it bouncing around from doctor to doctor. Unfortunately, the Endocrinologist also fails to find anything wrong with her nodule. With a deep sigh of defeat, the doctor said, "I'm sorry, but you're just going to need precautionary surgery to remove it. It's best to be proactive in the event that it is cancer."

This time, she felt fear take over her body. She looked

down at her round growing belly and said, "Can I really have major surgery while being this far along in my pregnancy?"

With confidence, the doctor said, "Of course you can! The baby will go to sleep with you."

My mother felt an odd sensation in her gut — and it wasn't me kicking. It was her intuition trying to tell her that this just didn't sound right. So, before she scheduled any surgery, she called her primary doctor and pediatrician to hear their thoughts. They both gave her the green light to go under the knife. With three doctors ensuring this would be safe, she scheduled her surgery at the front desk. She was just so ready for this to be over, and if that meant surgery, then fine. She had reached her wits' end and wanted her energy and vitality back so she could be a great mother to her babies. With eyelids as heavy as lead and a stomach growling from hunger for two, she mustered up every ounce of energy to drive home - to another baby waiting to be cared for.

———◆———

A month later, she wakes up before the sunrise feeling completely unrested as usual. Only this morning is extra rough - she hasn't eaten anything for eight hours and isn't allowed to do so before the big surgery to remove the nodule on her thyroid. Feeling like this can't be good for a woman who is 8-months into her pregnancy, her anxiety makes her wonder if the baby could be starving too? She quiets her thoughts at the reassurance of three doctors that this is a safe procedure. Within an hour, she's on the road to the hospital to get this over with. A single piece of toast is the only thing on her mind as she enters through the hospital doors and into a white gown. She's daydreaming of the huge meal she will eat after this is over as the nurse walks in to hook her up to an

IV. The nurse rolls her down the hallway on a stretcher into the pre-op room. It's go time.

The fluorescent lights are bright in this room; they accentuate the newfound stretch marks on her belly that has really popped in the last month. She sighs and waits for the anesthesiologist to come in.

Moments later a tall woman dressed in all white scrubs holding a clipboard walks in; it's the anesthesiologist. She reviews the process of anesthesia and prepares my mother for what to expect before and after the procedure. As she explains the countdown she will give her before she falls asleep, her attention promptly turns to a round belly poking out of the gown. Her pupils dilate.

"OH. You're...pregnant?" the doctor says, completely taken back.

Before my mom could answer, with a forced smile, the anesthesiologist says:

"Could you wait here one moment? I'll be right back."

She flees out of the room.

My mother instantly knew what this was about. She should've never scheduled a major surgery while this far along in her pregnancy. Her face flushes from anger and a hint of fear.

The anesthesiologist never returns. It was over an hour later when my mother, still sitting in the bright pre-op room, calls the nurse on her bedside phone to ask what was going on. The nurse says she will be right there and hangs up the phone. Before she gets to her bed, my mom sternly yells across the room, "Am I having surgery or not? I need to eat something!" The nurse denied her any food but agreed to at least unhook her from the IVs and remove her from the pre-op room. All thoughts of breakfast dissipated from my mother's head as the only words she could choke out were: What the fuck.

It is now over three hours since she arrived at the hospital. Surgery should have been over by now, but instead, multiple different anesthesiologists have walked in her room, took one look at her bulging belly, and walked right out. Adrenaline takes over her body and she sits up out of bed to dig in her purse and find her pediatrician's number. She frantically dials from her bedside phone. The receptionist answers and, after hearing my mother's situation, immediately transfers her to the doctor's emergency line.

"Didn't you say surgery while 8-months pregnant was fine? You told me this was ok!!" my mother shouts into the phone.

"Yes, everything should be okay. What's the issue?" said the pediatrician.

"Every anesthesiologist in this hospital refuses to put me under. No one will carry on with surgery. I haven't had a bite to eat in over 12 hours. Am I going to kill my baby if I go through with this?" she asks, her voice now cracking from tears.

The doctor is silent. Seconds pass before a nervous voice says, "I... I don't know what you should do. Let me speak with them first."

She hangs up the phone and waits yet another hour. No one calls her back or even comes in the room. She calls the nurse to declare she is leaving. They all agree she will not be having surgery today, but will need to come in immediately after birth to get this golf ball-sized mass removed.

It was a little over 30 days later on a cold Tuesday in December when my mother, with her long brown hair in a braid, walks into the same hospital. This time, with an optimistic energy, as she was about to meet her new baby. She never found out the gender, so today is extra exciting.

She's had vivid dreams of this baby being a boy, so she rubs her belly and talks to this 'curly haired boy named Nicholas that she's seen in many visions. She puts on the same white gown and, this time, makes her way to the birthing unit of the hospital. She brushes her braid away from the large red lump on her neck, as she's ready to forget everything else and focus solely on giving birth. Moments later, she is induced, and with a short labor and delivery… out comes a beautiful baby girl.

Feeling a surge of energy and vitality that she hasn't felt in years, she yells across the room to my father, "Chris! Look! She looks… well, *she* looks just like *me!*"

It's true. I have her eyes, her nose, and her long brown hair. Soon she'll see that I also have her endearing personality that she hasn't felt in years. She gives me the name Stephanie after her Yugoslavian grandmother, Stephana and, unable to let go of the Nicholas who visited her in many dreams… she declares my middle name to be Nicole.

She's home now, with her two babies and a new level of responsibility. A few days have passed and the newborn excitement has worn off since being home and back to reality. In between changing a toddler's diapers and breast feeding a newborn, she receives voicemails and letters from her endocrinologist inquiring about scheduling surgery. With an unsupportive husband rarely at home, she is taking on the daunting role of a single parent with two kids under two, so of course she hasn't scheduled surgery yet. One day after receiving the third letter asking her to schedule surgery, she goes to the bathroom to look in the mirror. Do I really need to do this? She questions. Her eyes widen with fear as she realizes the lump on her neck is no longer the size of a golf ball; it's doubled in size.

———◆———

It's been a month since she gave birth. She's approaching her 29th birthday and is ready to remove this lump so she can start a new chapter in life. She leaves her two babies with family and heads to the hospital. This time, without the pregnant belly scaring every anesthesiologist away, everything goes smoothly. The anesthesiologist counts backwards from 10, 9, 8, 7….

Before she knows it, she's waking up with a necklace shaped incision around her neck tied together with stitches. She's wondering how her babies are doing when the doctor walks in to tell her how well surgery went. The nodule was on its way to the lab to be tested for cancer and they should know within a few days. He sends her home to rest.

The very next day, my mother is jolted from her nap by the phone ringing. She answers with a soft, 'Hello?'

"Hi, may I speak with Lisa Powers?" the serious voice on the other end asks.

"Yes? This is she?" my mother says, more alert.

It's the Doctor. Her heart sinks because she can immediately sense his nervous energy. This can't be good news; why would he call so soon? With hesitation, he delivers the blow; the nodule was cancer. He urges her to come back in first thing tomorrow morning to have her entire thyroid removed. In his urgency, he forgot to mention she would be reliant on medication for the rest of her life. But it's the '80s, and cancer is so new and terrifying, that no one cares at this point. She schedules surgery for 8:00 the next morning.

It's five months later and the heat of the Midwest summer is intense. Every few weeks, my mother packs up my brother and me, and we make our way back to that same hospital where she gave new life and removed a tumor that was taking her own. This time not for surgery, but for required radiation treatment after the removal of her thyroid. She hauled a chunky baby on her hip while holding my brother's little hand as he walked by her side.

My grandma watches my brother and me in the waiting room while my mother goes into a special room for radiation. She is intimidated by this room; it feels more like a cage than a room for healing. It has no windows and the doors are very heavy. People walk in decked out in what appears to be space suits, holding a big metal capsule.

They unlock and unscrew it in front of my mother only to find another metal capsule in the previous one. Twist, twist unlock. Another capsule. Twist, twist unlock, one more capsule. Twist, twist, click! Finally. Her radioactive iodine pill is handed to her by a hand covered in a thick lead glove. She stares at the pill in astonishment; why would I ever put something this dangerous into my body? But, she trusts the doctor's orders and swallows it down with a big glass of tap water.

The radiation immediately gets to work, swarming her neck area to kill any remaining thyroid tissue. She doesn't feel anything as the doctor tells her she can get up to be released from her 'cage'. The heavy door closes tightly behind her, as my mother runs to me with a smile to pick me up. I'm still unable to hold my head up, so I fall into her neck and cuddle my way to comfort…right next to the radioactive iodine she just swallowed.

"This was my first taste of Healthcare in America."

—*Lisa Powers*

My Story

"**W**ould you like to schedule surgery to remove your thyroid now?"

How a routine pap smear turned into a doctor asking me if I wanted to remove one of the most vital organs in my body is still the most amazing thing to me; it was the catalyst behind why I pursued a profession as a health coach. The words in that question will echo in my head forever.

I was 25 years old and just moved from New Hampshire to a little town in South Carolina right outside of the big city, Charlotte, NC. I just married a boy I met in elementary school, too. We were both tired of the same routine, same people, and the cold weather was always such a drag. So, we quieted our minds and followed our intuition; we put a deposit down on an apartment we found online and left.

It's funny looking back because, in order to block the seeds of self-doubt being planted by friends and family, we lied and assured everyone we had jobs lined up in Charlotte. *We didn't. Sorry guys.* We not only moved down there with no jobs lined up, but we also moved down there with no bed, no furniture, and no idea what the future held. We were that ready for a new beginning.

It was a bit intimidating moving a thousand miles from home with no money or job. But we did it and, within a couple of weeks, we both had full-time jobs with benefits. The Universe always pulls through when you follow your intuition. Trust in that. Once our health insurance was set up, I decided to get all of my routine health visits done - find a new OBGYN, Dentist, PCP, the usual.

A few weeks later, I'm balancing a clipboard on my knee while filling out a health history form at one of the top-rated OBGYNs in my area. I'm watching pregnant women walk in and out for what feels like hours when they finally call my name. The nurse guides me down the hall and, instead of going into an exam room, she takes me to the doctor's personal office that looks more like a college professor's work space rather than a doctor's office. The OBGYN has requested to go over my entire health history before we begin the pap smear. The nurse assures me that the doctor will be right in and closes the door with a smile. Silence. I'm looking out the window and at all the photos of her and her family on the ledge. They all look so happy and healthy. And she's a dancer! Wow.

It feels like another hour goes by before the doctor finally walks in and introduces herself while apologizing for the wait. These poor doctors are stretched so thin. I don't complain about the long wait; my mom has been a nurse my whole life so I know just how busy these health professionals are. We dive right into my health history when she flips the page and reads the first line. Her eyes widen with concern.

"Your mother had thyroid cancer?" she asks, as she leans in closer, eyes fixed on mine waiting for a response.

She looks serious. No other doctor has ever questioned this on my health history. Why now? A wave of nervous energy takes over my body so I try to bring humor into the conversation. "Yes, all while she was pregnant with me. She even held me after her radioactive iodine treatments! Ha! Crazy, right?" I lightheartedly say.

She doesn't return the smile. In a serious tone, she orders, "Right after your pap smear, I want you to head down the hall to the right; we are going to get your labs done to check your thyroid today."

She didn't give me a chance to respond. This was definitely an order, not an option. Because I grew in a body that was growing cancer, I've had my thyroid checked routinely all my life, and it always checked out fine. But maybe this doctor knew something all the others didn't? After my pap smear and breast exam I walked down the hallway to get my blood drawn. I sit down and place my arm face up, ready for the dreaded smell of alcohol wipes.

The energy in the room is tense; I can tell the phlebotomist is wondering if I'm one of those people that pass out at the sight of needles, all while I'm wondering if my nervousness is making her nervous. So, again, I begin cracking jokes as she pierces my skin without warning and pulls four tubes of blood out of my arm. My comedic side quickly fades away when I stand up to leave and my knees buckle. Shit. I'm hit with the realization that it's been over four hours since I ate any food or even had a sip of water. I start to see black spots and the phlebotomist can see it in my pale face. She walks me to an empty exam room to rest with some pretzels and water.

Once I regained my strength, I walked out of that doctor's office with a growling stomach and white gauze taped tightly around my arm. It wasn't even five days later when I received a frantic call from the nurse.

"Is this Stephanie?" she quickly asked.

"Yes… this is she?" I slowly responded.

"Stephanie, we just received your lab work back and

your thyroid is VERY hyperthyroid. We need to refer you to a specialist right away."

She seemed very concerned. Although I wasn't at first, I absorbed her energy and became really nervous too. I barely remember her explaining what 'hyperthyroid' meant and how confusing it was to distinguish hypo from hyper. But I remember the words cancer, goiter, medication, and surgery being thrown around. Having no idea what hyperthyroid meant, I asked her to please clarify. She read my lab result to me: 0.053 TSH, which means my thyroid is producing too many hormones. I was so confused, because to me that number seemed low which would indicate hypothyroid...but apparently, it's just the opposite.

The nurse had already scheduled my visit to an endocrinologist before we hung up. This time it would be to get my labs drawn again but also to get an ultrasound of my thyroid. I was afraid, confused, and totally caught off guard so, without question, I obliged to go. Before we hung up, I asked her why it is that my thyroid could be so off balance when I felt just fine? After a pause, she said, "The endocrinologist will be able to tell you more" and hung up.

Little did I know at the time, my definition of 'just fine' was not normal...

———◆———

It's a month later when I'm sitting in the office of the endocrinologist holding my husband's hand while diabetic sock commercials played overhead on the TV. We are the youngest ones in the building by far. The nurse calls me back and we make our way to the exam room. They take all of my vitals and explain the procedure of the day - an ultrasound of my neck to ensure my thyroid isn't enlarged. They were also going to draw my labs to check my thyroid levels again, and this time check for antibodies. Anti-what? I thought. Oh well, these guys are professionals — they know what they're doing. Moments later, a beautiful girl around my age rolls in a cart with the ultrasound machine on it and turns off the lights. She applies a cool gel over my neck and gently places the scanner on it, slowly moving back and forth. Her eyes are squinting at the screen as she stalls on my left side for a little while. She excuses herself to go grab the doctor. *Uh oh*, I think. The doctor comes in and squints his eyes at the screen too.

"Hmm…No, no that's nothing. I think it's just anatomy." the doctor says, almost under his breath.

I look up at the nurse and ask if they found something wrong. Without moving her eyes to look at me, she continues staring at the ultrasound screen while explaining they thought my thyroid was enlarged but it turns out it's just my anatomy. I apparently just have a large thyroid gland. She wipes the excess gel off my neck and packs up her equipment. Moments later, the doctor comes back in and flips on the lights. He says he has good news and bad news. The good news is, my thyroid does not have any nodules or tumors growing on it. The bad news is, according to my labs from the OBGYN, I have hyperthyroidism which is going to make naturally conceiving a baby next to impossible and come with many complications.

I'm staring at the ground as he's going over the list of common symptoms and future complications hyperthyroidism can cause. Anxiety, heart palpitations, infertility, thyroid storm…his words begin to fade as my mouth curves into a strange smile, almost out of my control. I have no idea where it came from, but something inside of me just knew all of this was not….real. I somehow intuitively knew that this issue was easily preventable and reversible, yet here the doctor was giving me the worse case scenarios and asking me if I wanted to try radiation therapy to kill my thyroid or schedule surgery to remove it. I snap back into reality.

He looks up from his notes and directly at me for an answer.

"Would you like to schedule surgery to remove your thyroid now?" he repeats.

"Doctor, thank you for all of that information. Could you tell me anything I should change with my diet or lifestyle that might help this?"

He is completely taken back by this question. I can tell no one has asked it before. After a few moments of thinking, he says, "No, not really, this is just a genetic thing... but, uh, eat more kale?" He said with an unconfident tone. I can tell he knows more than he feels he is allowed to say... perhaps he feels too liable to tell the truth. He immediately changes the subject to remind me to stop by the lab to get my blood drawn, then leaves.

I turn to my husband with a look of *'what the hell just happened?'* only to find a similar look on his face. We grab our stuff and walk to the lab to get my blood drawn again.

A week later, I receive an email from the Endocrinologist stating my lab results were in. I anxiously log into my online portal to read the results:

TSH: Normal

T3: Normal

T4: Normal

Thyroid Antibodies: High

Underneath my results was a little note from the doctor explaining that my labs all came back normal besides for my thyroid antibodies.They were elevated at 45, which indicates I'm in the beginning stages of an autoimmune disease called Hashimotos Thyroiditis. He tells me to research it and call him with any questions. He continues to explain that because the rest of my thyroid results are fine, that I do not need to come in for a follow-up. If I intend to get pregnant in the next few months, however, to come see him.

As I read this new diagnosis, I have so many emotions vibrating through me. What the hell is Hashimotos? What are thyroid antibodies? I have an autoimmune disease? Whatever happened to being hyperthyroid? How could that one nurse tell me my thyroid was so out of whack but then, a month later, it's normal? None of this was adding up.

It was time to become my own best doctor and take charge of my health.

———◆———

Growing in a womb that was growing cancer, it almost seems inevitable that I would have a thyroid issue upon birth. Strangely, I did not; my thyroid labs always came back normal. It wasn't until I was 25 years old that I would develop any issue with my thyroid - right around the same time my mother started to have an issue with hers. My mother was 28 when she was diagnosed with thyroid cancer. I am 28 and writing a book on how to prevent it. The Universe works in such mysterious ways...

I truly feel lucky that I dodged that bullet. I easily could have been undergoing the same thyroid surgery as my mom, at the same age too. It breaks my heart when my mom asks, "Where was this book when I was your age?" While I couldn't save her, I can give you all of the tools you need to heal yourself. Diet and lifestyle changes paired with deep emotional healing are ultimately what led me to the reversal of my Hashimotos Thyroid Disease. Emotional healing probably playing the biggest role. It should be noted that almost all people who are diagnosed with an autoimmune disease have gone through a traumatic event in their life; most commonly right before their diagnosis. You'll find out in Chapter 3 what traumatic event happened to me.

Whenever the inevitable writer's block creeps in to disrupt the writing process, I like to think of my mother holding a copy of this book in her hands at 28 years old. Perhaps, if she had read Thyroid First Aid Kit, she could've healed herself without a drastic surgery. How different her experience with motherhood could have been…

I wish I could go back and communicate with her through the womb, so I could tell her to leave that plastics factory and never look back. I wish I could tell her to use a little less of that drugstore lotion next time she's getting ready for the day. Mostly, I wish I could communicate to her the importance of speaking her truth. I suppose this book is fulfilling that wish.

My only hope by writing the Thyroid First Aid Kit is that some woman, whether she's a teenager struggling with self-image issues, a young mother wondering how she'll ever get through this, or an older woman looking to feel a lust for life again… I just hope this book finds her and helps her get back to who she longs to be. Same for my male readers! I hope this book provides you with reassurance that what you're feeling — from the symptoms of your disease to the frustration & anxiety of multiple doctor visits — that's something we are all experiencing together.

If you're reading this book because your thyroid disease has made you hit rock bottom, then I'm here to tell you that that's a great place to be — because now, there's nowhere to go but up.

Let's begin.

CHAPTER 1
Gluten Free Guru

*You aren't allergic to wheat; you're allergic
to the way we grow it.*

Isn't it odd that people are becoming deathly allergic
to staple foods such as bread or pasta? What is gluten
anyway? *Gluten is the substance added to wheat products
to make them soft and chewy.*

I'll never forget last October when I walked by the
Halloween candy aisle at Target and saw an entire row
dedicated to Gluten Free candy. I wondered what my grandparents would think of this. Throughout my career as a health
coach, I have heard countless people claim there's no way
they can have a wheat allergy, as their family was raised on
pizza and pasta and cereals. If their parents and grandparents
never had an issue with it… why would they get the short
end of the stick?

Well, you aren't really allergic to wheat. You are allergic
to the way we grow it today. When our grandparents ate
wheat, they were eating conventionally grown wheat —
grown organically in tune with nature. Today, through

genetic engineering, we grow wheat double the size and harvest double the amount. We also use a hefty amount of chemicals to keep our crops looking perfect and bug free. The most common pesticide used on wheat is a chemical called Glyphosphate. Once a bug consumes even the slightest bit of this chemical, they explode. If this chemical makes bugs explode, what does it do to our stomachs when we eat it?

Gluten affects people on different levels; it's a very bio-individual substance. For some people, the symptoms are so mild that they go unnoticed for years. For others, the symptoms can be as serious as vomiting, diarrhea, and hospitalization. I'll never forget an acquaintance sharing her story of how she figured out she had Celiac Disease. She drove to a friend's house for a party one weekend and ate pizza while she was there. On her way home, she felt 'funny' and had digestive upset.

Figuring it was just the cheese on the pizza, she continued driving home. The funny feeling intensified. She eventually became so dizzy that she fainted at the wheel. The ER never for a minute imagined it could be from gluten, so they hooked her up to IVs to replenish electrolytes and sent her home. This fainting continued on for weeks until someone finally mentioned that her symptoms sounded like a severe wheat allergy. She immediately eliminated gluten from her diet and, within one day, she was back to normal. Weeks later, she found out through a test of her stomach lining that she indeed had Celiac Disease.

For me, gluten tore up my gut lining and caused a host of long-term issues, specifically fatigue and severe allergies. The sad part is I had no clue for years; I always thought bloat and fatigue were something everyone experienced. Up next, I'm going to share with you exactly how I discovered I had an allergy to wheat. I didn't see it coming; I always thought that was one allergy I would never have. But the clues were always RIGHT in front of me for years. Hopefully this book will help you identify if you, too, are suffering from a gluten allergy.

———◆———

The vibration of my Nokia cellphone wakes me up. It's my alarm getting me up for high school. Ugh, will I ever get enough sleep? As the orange glow of the sunrise begins to illuminate my room, I immediately regret how late I went to bed last night. Oh — here it comes. I flinch my nose and scrunch my face in pain. Every single morning, I get this awful 'pins & needles' sensation up in my sinuses. The best way to describe this daily occurrence is the same sensation you get when soda or chlorine goes up your nose.

Shortly after, I fall into a sneezing fit and sneeze so many times in a row that I get chest pain. Everyone in my house is now up and getting ready for their day due to my loud sinus eruptions. I'm like a guaranteed alarm clock for them. I walk downstairs to greet everyone with eyes so puffy I can barely see.

"Geeeesh," my mom says looking at me, as I blow my red nose. This has been my routine for years, I can't believe she's still surprised by this.

"Just another day," I mutter in a raspy voice as I reach for the last tissue in the Kleenex box. I go through at least one box a week. Two in the spring.

I'll never forget the day I discovered I had allergies. I was a 10-year-old tomboy wearing black soccer shorts and a white t-shirt with the Earth on it, only, the Earth wasn't all ocean and land — but covered in all of the animals of the world. Deer, giraffes, rhinos, lions, birds, reptiles. This shirt was discolored and worn out with small holes starting to form. I loved animals more than anything in the world and if I got to wear them all on a shirt, even better. I had just moved north to New Hampshire from my home of Southern Indiana. We were out exploring our new city when I asked my mom to stop at a local pet store. She knew very well about my love for animals, so she obliged.

I anxiously run into the store to discover I hit the jackpot; KITTENS. I stick my dirty fingers through the cage to pet them. I put my nose to theirs and eventually sweet talked my way into holding one. There was one all black kitten that reminded me of my cat I just left behind in Indiana, Sylvia. I immediately fall in love. While my mom was with my brother looking at lizards, I cuddled this kitten to my neck and hummed her a song. The kitten started to purr and I felt happier than I had in weeks since our big move. I had to adjust this kitten a lot so I could reach my neck to scratch it, but I just figured it was her whiskers tickling me.

I hear my mom yell from the front of the store, "Stephanie! Let's go!" I opened the cage and put the kitten back with her litter. I ran out of the store and jumped into the back seat of our old Dodge Caravan.

I was still scratching my neck, but now also my cheeks. My face felt hot and swollen, and I was starting to feel my pulse in my cheeks. We're silently driving down the road when I catch my mom's green eyes looking back at mine through the rearview mirror. They grow wide with shock.

"STEPHANIE NICOLE. Whats wrong!?" She yells back at me. Everyone turns to look.

"Well, my face is a little itchy mommy," I quietly say.

She immediately pulls the van over and tells me to get out. She grabs my chin and forcefully moves my head back and forth as she examines my cheeks, lips, and neck. I'm covered in welts and hives from my chest up. We pile back into the van and speed to a CVS drugstore. She prompts me to get out of our red van and grabs my hand as we rush into the store. She purchases a box of allergy pills and breaks one in half. They are a pretty pink color, so I happily agree to swallow one. She rubs a cool cream on my rashes and they immediately feel better.

I didn't think much of it.

I grew up running around the fields of Southern Indiana. Animals, and all the germs they come with, were a part of my every day barefoot routine. Most of my baby photos feature me spooning with dogs or carrying big barn cats the same size as me. Days were spent rolling in the grass and building forts in corn fields. I don't recall sneezing once in those eight years. How could this just develop?

As soon as we've settled into our home in New Hampshire, I find myself with my mom at an appointment with our new doctor. My mom mentions the pet store episode to the doctor and she instantly refers me to an allergist for testing. The doctor turns to me and gently explains that my allergy tests will involve a lot of needles. I wasn't thrilled.

My day with the allergist came quicker than I would have preferred. The doctor didn't waste any time — she came walking in with the needle packs and showed me what allergen each needle contained. This was a pack of about eight small needles, each containing a common allergen. One was oak, the other was grass. One held dog dander while the one next to it had cat. When she mentioned cat and dog dander, my stomach sank at the thought of being allergic to the thing I love most in this world.

The allergist instructed me to lay down on my belly with my shirt off. I hate the sound of that crackling paper. The smell of alcohol wipes filled the room as my mom stood in the corner looking nervous but stern. The doctor stood over me with the needle pack lightly balanced on my back, and gave me to the count of three. Liar. Before she said three she forcefully put her weight on the needle pack and eight needles pierced my skin at once. I clenched my eyes so tight tears squeezed out of the cracks. She ripped it out and prepared for the second pack. As she rubbed the other side of my back with alcohol wipes, the worst burning sensation raged through my body. It felt like someone lit a fire on my back. Under the assumption that me not saying anything meant I was okay, she shoved the second needle pack into my back without a countdown.

As the doctor starts to clean up, she tells me to relax but focus on any itchy spots, and to let my mom know which ones hurt. They all hurt lady, I think to myself. But there were two that itched so bad I grew a lump in my throat out of frustration of not being able to scratch them. I pointed them out to my mom and begged her to rub her nails against them.

"The two at the bottom. Yes the ones right next to each other. Those itch so bad like nothing I've ever felt before. Please just touch them!!" I begged.

"Uh oh, I think those two are the cat and dog dander," My mom said.

My heart sank. *No No No. Please don't be animals. If this doctor walks in and tells me I'm allergic to cats and dogs....* tears start rolling down my red cheeks.

The doctor walks in and examines my welts. She begins checking off boxes on my medical record:

- ❑ Grass
- ❑ Pollen
- ❑ Dust
- ❑ Cat
- ❑ Dog

And just like that, I was diagnosed as being allergic to cats and dogs. When the doctor delivered the tragic news to me, my sadness morphed into anger. How dare this woman in her fancy white coat tell me not to hold cats or pet dogs anymore. Like a hormonal teenager I looked at her and told her I would never stop playing with animals. She could sense my passion and urged me to just think about it. I didn't budge. She then explained the dander I'm allergic to is mostly on cat whisker pores and in dog's mouths. At this point, it was in one ear and out the other; my thoughts revolved around WHY ME? I was notorious for being an animal lover. Now I can't go near them? Something is not natural about this. We are made to be surrounded by nature, not allergic to it — and I knew this at 10 years old.

Before the doctor handed us a prescription, she explained to me how serious allergies can get. She said that if I did not take my daily medicine or avoid my allergens that I may need steroid shots just to be able to breathe. My mom scheduled a follow up appointment to test for asthma and refill my prescription. It was from this day forward that I took allergy pills every single day for over a decade...

———◆———

I'm now a junior in high school and thank goodness I don't have a full schedule of classes. Today, I just so happen to have a couple of hours in-between school and my job working in the kitchen at a local hospital. Score. The thought of taking a nap before work was all the motivation I needed to pull me out of bed to get ready for the day.

I spend way too much time burning CDs rather than making breakfast, so I rush out the door to try to get to school on time. Hungry, I pull into our local Dunkin' Donuts and grab a quick breakfast consisting of an untoasted bagel with strawberry cream cheese and a strawberry Coolata with whipped cream spilling over the top. I throw my bagel in my backpack and turn up the bass to wake up. Nothing like a little Jay-Z at seven in the morning.

I get to my first class of the day and take out my bagel. I smother all the cream cheese on both slices leaving nothing to spare. I try my best to pay attention for the rest of class, but 20 minutes into the lecture my eyes are rolling back. The little energy I have is being used towards trying my best to stay awake; never mind absorbing the information being taught to us.

By second period, its a little after 10:00 a.m. Despite sitting front row, my eyes cannot stay open for the life of me. I can feel my eyelids start to weigh 20lbs each and my eyeballs become so dry. Damn it. Why am I always so tired! I can sense that my teacher now notices. Sometimes these sleepy sessions get so intense that I have to go to the bathroom just to walk it off or splash water on my face. My mom tells me I've been this way since I was a little girl and, to an extent, she's right. Ever since I could talk, I have needed a nap at 3:00 in the afternoon and always get tired before my friends. She thinks it's cute and I just accept it as 'genetic.'

———◆———

Almost a decade goes by before I discover the true root of my 3 p.m. crash. After I graduate college in 2011, I start to hear a lot about this 'gluten-free' fad — my mom even bought gluten free bread once to try it out. It was the most disgusting, cardboard-tasting bread I've ever had. It crumbled to pieces the moment I picked it up. Who eats this stuff?! These fad diets are so weird. I figured this was just another phase like Weight Watchers or South Beach Diet; it will pass.

Besides, being allergic to wheat would never happen to me. No way. I may be allergic to animals and plants, but bread? Ha. Nope. I was never one of those kids deathly allergic to a simple food, carrying around an epi-pen incase someone had a peanut butter sandwich. I loved my bagels and pretzels. My favorite part of pizza was the crust. When I started dating my Sicilian husband, there was nothing that made me feel more loved than when he made me homemade alfredo pasta and garlic bread.

In 2014, I started to experience something else besides fatigue: severe bloating. I'll never forget the day my mom and I were touring Charleston, SC when I ate a lox bagel for breakfast. A few hours later, I was too tired to continue our tour of a plantation, and my stomach was protruding so much it hurt. I went to the bathroom in our hotel room to let my gut hang out in front of the mirror to see just how bad it was. As I stared in the mirror both angry and in disbelief, I could feel my skin stretching like I was pregnant.

'Something is so wrong,' I thought.

The following year, through divine synchronicity, I figured out what was wrong. I was visiting Colorado for the first time with my husband. We were staying at the coolest Airbnb — the Halean Lifestream Center in Crestone, Colorado. It's owned by a trauma surgeon turned holistic doctor, Dr. John Day. As he's giving us a tour of the place, he mentions he has an inversion table in his office. Excited, I ask if we can go in and see it. He unlocks the door to his office and we follow him in.

I'm instantly intrigued by all of the holistic books and photos in his office. My husband and I walk around, stopping to read things on the wall as if we were in a museum. There's one black and white photo of his family with Helen Keller that I break the silence to ask him about.

"Oh, my mother was her doctor," he casually says.

I look over at my husband who looks just as astonished as I do and mouth a big 'WOW' as Dr.John is digging around a closet for the inversion table. We all eventually gravitate to his desk and I sit across from him to chat. We're talking about the state of health in America when I interrupt him to say 'Oh yeah! And tell me why so many women have a thyroid issue nowadays? I was just diagnosed with Hashimotos last year.'

He doesn't respond. He looks at me with thinking eyes and eventually says, "You need to eliminate grains." He slides his chair back to dig through his desk drawers. He's sifting through a folder of papers when he finally pulls one out. He slides it across the desk over to me:

- ❏ Wheat
- ❏ Corn
- ❏ Soy
- ❏ Rice

I look back up at him with a confused face. He leans back in his chair and folds his hands together.

"You have leaky gut syndrome. Everyone with a thyroid or autoimmune condition has leaky gut," he says with calm confidence.

I scrunch my face to show disgust. Leaky gut? That sounds...so gross.

"What exactly does that mean?" I ask in a faint tone.

"It simply means your gut lining is inflamed and has holes in it. Foods, especially grains, are only adding to the problem. All of the food you eat is escaping through the holes in your gut wall and entering your bloodstream. Your body mistakes these food particles as invaders and attacks itself, especially the thyroid gland."

I look down at the paper, then up at Dr.John. I look over at my husband who seems just as clueless as me. I think about the delicious bag of pretzels I just bought at Trader Joe's, waiting for me in my backpack over at the house.

"So, I need to go on the gluten-free diet?" I ask, nervous for his response.

"Yes. Completely gluten-free," Dr. John says

My heart sinks. Dr.John's blue eyes were very serious and, despite having just met him, I felt as though he cared about my health more than any white coat doctor I've ever been in contact with. I could feel the sincerity in his words and knew it was time for me to completely clean up my diet. I had to go all or nothing, or else this autoimmune disease would take over. Then it hit me: *I'm on vacation. I like to eat whatever I want when I'm on vacation! Shit.*

I walked back to our room, feeling a bit upset, sifting through thoughts of: *what the hell will I eat for breakfast in the morning? Bagel? Nope. Toast? Not happening. Cereal? Cant have it. What am I supposed to eat!?* Before I even take off my shoes, I unzip my green backpack and dig to the bottom for my Trader Joe's pretzels. I turn them around to read the ingredients list. First ingredient: Enriched Wheat Flour. With regret, for both my wallet and my taste buds, I toss them in the trash and make my way to bed with my tail between my legs.

I wake up the next morning still feeling defeated, wondering how on earth I'm going to pull this off. No bagel? No cereal? What am I supposed to eat around here? I'm going to starve. We were in a tiny town at the base of a mountain in the middle of nowhere. My favorite thing to do while on vacation is go out for breakfast. Mitch reassures me that I could always just get scrambled eggs somewhere. Great.

We head into town and stop at the only café — a vintage style eatery attached to a tiny grocery; the only grocery in town. We walk past locals smoking cigarettes outside and make our way in. Immediately, we feel like elephants in the room as everyone's eyes maneuver to us. Everyone is dressed in worn, gypsy style clothing, yet working on thousand-dollar Mac Books. I assume they're all locals wondering who we are and how two young tourists found Crestone. I feel like I'm on a runway as I walk up to the counter and look up at their menu on a chalkboard above the register. A dusty star in the corner of the black chalkboard catches my eye as I read:

*Note: All items served Gluten Free.

What!?!

I turn around and look at Mitch with wide eyes.

"Look! I can get a breakfast sandwich! Or Avocado toast!!" I clap like a child, not caring what the audience of locals thought of my excitement.

I was so excited to order whatever I wanted without restrictions, that the memory of my mom's gluten-free cardboard bread fell out of my memory. I ordered a breakfast sandwich and it ended up being the best sandwich I've ever had. After breakfast, we went to the tiny grocery attached to the café to buy some stuff for the Airbnb; my new diet called for lots of cooking at home. We ended up making the most delicious, vegetable filled, gluten/grain free meal for dinner that night. It was fun being in the kitchen together and eating under the stars in a dining room made out of all windows. It was just the two of us in silence; no waiters, no crowds or loud noises from a bar. I didn't even get bloated after eating! This diet wasn't so bad after all.

On the day we had to make our way back to Denver to fly home, we drove by a tiny coffee shop just outside of Crestone. We walked in to grab a couple of coffees when a jolly woman standing next to a display of freshly baked muffins greets us. I began ordering but had to stop myself to make a comment about the homemade muffins.

"It's too bad I just started a gluten-free diet, otherwise I would order all of those muffins!" I said with a giggle.

"Honey, that's all we have are gluten-free muffins," the woman said with a 'welcome to the new age' smile.

I walked out of that coffee shop and into the desert carrying a coffee and a bag full of the rest of her blueberry muffins.

———◆———

It was a week later when I woke up at home with my two cats resting at my feet. Bright Carolina sun poking through the blinds. I threw the covers off to get my day started. As I began my morning routine it dawned on me…I walked right past the almost empty tissue box on my nightstand to go to the bathroom. I even went all the way to the kitchen to feed the cats without sneezing once! Could it be…?

As I'm standing in front of the bathroom mirror brushing my teeth, I realize, for the first time in probably my entire life, I don't have puffy circles around my eyes. My complexion actually looks amazing! I lean in closer to the mirror: my eyes aren't red! I don't have dark bags under them! I run to share the breaking news with my husband.

"Yeah, I was just about to say something. I've noticed you haven't sneezed at all since we got home from Colorado!" He said to me with excitement.

A Christmas miracle. My ego wanted to tell me that it was just a lucky day or maybe it's just the cooler weather. Just last month I couldn't comprehend waking up without blowing my nose. I had only been gluten-free for one week, and in that short time my allergies went away, my eyes were bright and my skin was clear. By week two, my stomach was flatter than I've ever seen it. By week three, I stopped getting tired every afternoon and by week four, I stopped drinking coffee. A dear friend once told me that gluten free is like wearing rose colored glasses; you have no idea what great health feels like until you eliminate it.

After week 4 I began researching foods to help patch up the holes in a leaky gut. More on that later in this chapter.

———◆———

It's a year later and I'm still gluten free. I left my home in Charlotte to start a new chapter in Charleston, South Carolina. As I always do when I move, I immediately schedule a visit with a new Primary Care Doctor to establish a relationship. I do the usual hour long stay in the waiting room before they call me back. As the doctor reviews my health history of hyperthyroid and Hashimotos, she was surprised at my reversal of the thyroid antibodies. She looked down at my record, then up at me, then down at my record again.

"How did you do this?" she curiously asked.

"I eliminated gluten from my diet," I nervously said, not expecting her to believe me.

"What? Like, you don't eat bread or pizza or anything?" she said.

I laughed and told her I still eat all of that - just healthier versions. She seemed skeptical. I thought this would be a funny story to share with my friends and family. But as I walked out of her office and into a thunderstorm brewing outside, I wondered how many women she's prescribed lifetime thyroid medication to, when all they needed was a simple change of diet.

I sat in my car to pause and meditate on that sad notion. If I could just somehow get the message out to the masses, thyroid issues wouldn't be an epidemic like it is. Giant rain drops break the silence as they start hitting the roof of my car.

I'm too focused on the weight of my thoughts to give it any attention. If I could reverse my thyroid disease, anyone could do it. How come doctors don't know about gluten? Or leaky gut? People out there need to know this! I need to come up with a way to present it clearly and easily. Lightning flashes in my rearview mirror followed by ear piercing thunder. And in the midst of the rumble it hit me

Thyroid First Aid Kit.

The point of going Gluten-Free is to heal damage to the gut lining. Remember, wheat alone does not cause this damage. It is the chemicals we use to grow the wheat today that causes this. I have heard many people with Celiac Disease say they are able to eat all the pasta and bread they want overseas in places like Italy or Spain with zero side effects. This is because international countries still grow their wheat conventionally, without the use of heavy pesticides and genetic modification.

Will you have to go gluten-free forever? No. A good rule of thumb when figuring out how long you will need to stick with this lifestyle is: How long did it take you to develop a wheat allergy? For me that was years. I developed severe allergies, which were the first sign of damage to my gut lining, at age 10. So, I like to think I need to stick with a gluten-free diet for 10 years. I am on year three of being gluten-free and honestly have no plan of ever turning back.

Between getting rid of my severe allergies and gaining all this natural energy, it's second nature to go out to eat and ask for a sandwich to be wrapped in lettuce instead of a bun. My tastebuds now prefer it! The gluten free diet gives your body a chance to heal itself; to patch up holes in the gut lining.

I still eat avocado toast for breakfast and pizza for dinner, I just make it all at home with gluten-free ingredients.

If this is your first time going gluten-free, you're in luck! We've come a long way from the cardboard bread days back in 2010. There are so many delicious gluten-free options today. Many people have adopted the Gluten-Free diet because of health issues, and the food industry is supplying for the demand. There are several gluten-free options at nearly every grocery chain, and even popular restaurants are catering to this need. Note: You will typically find gluten-free bread in the freezer section! Not the regular bread aisle.

Most importantly, while you're eliminating gluten from your diet, you need to add in healing foods that rebuild the stomach lining. I'll share examples of these foods in the summary below. The more gut-friendly foods you eat, the faster your stomach lining will heal itself, and the quicker you can eat organic wheat products again.

Gluten Free Guru Summary:

What is Gluten?

The sticky substance that keeps bread products moist and intact.

Why can't I eat it?

Because the way we grow it in the USA is poisonous. We use a strong pesticide called Glyphosphate that makes bugs explode when they consume it. We consume Glyphosphate when we eat wheat, so if it makes bugs explode, what could it be doing to our stomachs? We've also genetically modified wheat so dramatically that we now grow twice as much, twice as fast. Our bodies cannot keep up with this genetically modified food.

How come my parents never had an issue with it?

Wheat was grown completely differently just a couple decades ago. Your parents are used to consuming conventionally grown wheat. Millennials are the first generation to be raised almost solely on pesticide covered, genetically modified food... and look at us. We are suffering from IBS and autoimmune diseases in our 20s. We have infertility clinics on every block. And when we do conceive a baby, they are born with several food allergies and digestive issues of their own.

How do I know I have a wheat allergy?

Research shows that nearly everyone diagnosed with a thyroid disorder has a connection to leaky gut, which is a direct connection to gluten sensitivity. Eliminate it from your diet and see how you feel. I didn't have the slightest clue that my allergies and 3 p.m. crash were due to pretzels...

In my health coach experience, a lot of people with wheat allergies have 'chicken skin' on the back of their arms and almost always experience bloating and/or fatigue after eating wheat.

Next time you eat something like pancakes or cereal for breakfast, try not drinking coffee and see if you can make it through the day without a nap. If you get so tired that you cant keep your eyes open, you probably have a wheat allergy.

What is leaky gut syndrome?

It is when someone has a tarnished gut lining, where tiny holes are created through a series of things like poor diet, gluten, toxins, strong drugs like antibiotics, and stress. It is still a grey area for medical professionals, so the chances of your doctor diagnosing you with it or even having knowledge of it are very slim. This is one topic I urge you to do lots of personal research on beyond this book.

What are the symptoms of leaky gut?

- ❑ Thyroid Conditions
- ❑ Autoimmune Conditions
- ❑ Mood Disorders
- ❑ Bloating
- ❑ Food Intolerances
- ❑ Acne

❑ Fatigue
❑ Headaches
❑ Digestive issues

What foods should I avoid?

❑ Wheat
❑ Dairy
❑ Sugar
❑ Grains

Note: Remember, everything is bio-individual. Some of these foods may be fine in your digestive system while others may not. I suggest starting with an elimination diet. Start by eliminating all of these food groups at once. Begin adding in each food group a week at a time to see which ones cause a reaction.

That said, I still believe everyone with a thyroid issue should eliminate gluten.

What foods will help repair leaky gut?

The following foods were a staple in my daily diet while I was healing my gut:

Kombucha:

This probiotic, fizzy tea is loaded with 'good bacteria' to help regulate digestion. I have had many clients cure their acid reflux just by drinking one of these a day!

My favorite brand is GT's Synergy because they do not add any excess sugar. You can find it everywhere from Whole Foods to Walmart.

Caution: Do not shake a kombucha. They will explode!

You can also home-brew your own to save money.

Bone Broth:

Loaded with the best vitamins and minerals for optimal gut health, bone broth is packed with collagen, which are the building blocks to patching up holes in the gut lining. Whole Foods now sells bone broth by the bottle as a grab-and-go option. A lot of people make their own at home. The best bones are from local farmers, or you can ask the deli at your local grocery for bones. Lots of recipes on Google or Pinterest! A sure-fire way to know if you made good bone broth is if it turns to jelly when refrigerated.

Fermented Foods:

Sauerkraut, organic pickles, pickled vegetables, etc. These foods, like kombucha, colonize the gut with good bacteria helping the lining of your stomach become thick and strong again.

Probiotic:

I recommend taking one-a-day to help re-colonize your gut to have more good bacteria than bad. I love the brand Udo's Choice by FLORA because it is human based probiotics rather than plant based. Our bodies react to and accept this type of good bacteria the best.

Dr.Axe also makes a great Leaky Gut Formula supplement. Google it! It's always out of stock, and for good reason - it contains every mineral you need to heal a leaky gut lining

What about pizza, bread, and pasta?

As I mentioned earlier, I still eat avocado toast and healthy, gluten-free versions of pizza. In my household, we love Trader Joe's gluten-free flour and make our own pizza crusts at home. We've also tried cauliflower crust! I love the brand 'Food for Life' for gluten-free toast — their black rice bread from Whole Foods is amazing! (You can find it in the freezer section.) A tried and true favorite brand of many gluten-free families is Udi's. They make wonderful breads and muffins that nearly mimic the consistency of gluten. Arrowhead Mills and Bobs Red Mills are two other great brands for making gluten-free baked goods at home. When I'm craving chocolate chip cookies, I use a popular social media vegan, Earthy Andy's, vegan/gluten free chocolate chip cookie recipe. No one ever knows they're vegan, in fact, people often comment that they are the best cookies they've ever had!

As for pasta, that one is so easy to replicate nowadays. At any grocery store you can find brown rice pasta in the regular pasta aisle. The texture and flavor is exactly the same, and, bonus: it cooks in half the time!

Note: There is growing evidence that gluten-free diets aren't actually as healthy as our society makes it out to be. This is because gluten-free products usually consist of a lot of starches like potato, white rice or tapioca that can spike our blood sugar. Eating gluten-free is not your new way of life. Until we can resort back to the conventional way of growing wheat here in the USA, and until you heal your leaky gut, I highly suggest sticking with it.

Heal your gut lining to heal your thyroid!

CHAPTER 2
Maybe she's born with it. Maybe it's her endocrine system.

'Genes load the gun, lifestyle pulls the trigger.'

—*Caldwell Esselstyn*

While eliminating gluten and moving to a more plant based diet showed immediate improvements to my health, in the long run, it was eliminating the daily toxins I was infusing into my body that played the biggest role in regaining balance to my hormones. Hours of personal research led to the startling conclusion that every day, women slather on upwards of 200+ chemicals before they even head out the door in the morning! Hairspray, makeup, deodorant, perfumes, lotions, soaps. Our bodies cannot possibly keep up with all of these toxins from both food and environment.

Before I even enrolled as a student at the Institute for Integrative Nutrition, I discovered a cutting-edge app for my iPhone that really played a pivotal role in my healing journey. It's called Think Dirty and it grades bathroom/household products on a scale of 1-10. A zero is ideal, which means it's a perfectly clean product for you to use in your home or on your body. If a product rates a 10 though, that indicates it should have a warning label on it that says: WARNING. INGREDIENTS IN THIS PRODUCT CAUSE CANCER.

The app breaks the ingredients down into three categories:

- **Carcinogenicity**
- **Developmental & Reproductive toxicity**
- **Allergies & Immunotoxicities**

To see just how toxic a product is, simply scan the barcode on its packaging using the Think Dirty app and wait a few seconds. A number grade will pop up, followed by a Dirty Meter and an ingredients list explaining why. Open the ingredients list and you'll see each individual ingredient rated on a scale of 1-10.

Let's use me as an example. I used to rub Garnier Skin Renew Anti-Puff Eye Roller around my eyes every single morning. I was convinced that I would look terrible throughout the day if I ever skipped an application. That green little tube was my lifesaver. When I scan this product, it rates an 8. When I look at the ingredients tab to see why, it states:

Imidazolidinyl Urea: "Urea allows chemicals to penetrate deeper into the skin, and is added to products as a preservative and anti-microbial. Urea can increase your risk for contact dermatitis, and has also been shown to release formaldehyde - a carcinogen."

Methylparaben: "Fragrance ingredient. Preservative, mimic estrogen and can act as a potential hormone system disruptor. (Some studies of breast tumors show a build-up of methylparabens in the breast tissue.)"

...and that's only two ingredients out of several more. I'll never forget the day I discovered Think Dirty and had a mini meltdown in my bathroom. I was scanning everything from my shampoo, conditioner, deodorant, lotion, and they all rated an 8 or higher. I opened my makeup bag to find the same thing - every product rated a 9 or higher. All had the phrase 'Hormone System Disruptor' attached to their ingredients.

How could they sell this stuff to us? Did I just discover the reason why so many women have thyroid issues? My mind started to go deep as I recalled every single chemical that's ever been absorbed by my body. Johnson&Johnson when I was a baby. (Rates a 9!) All the heavily scented detangler spray my mom used on my ratty hair as a kid. (Rates a 10!) All the cucumber melon scented lotions from high school. (Rates a 10!)

My head was spinning.

I would wake up and wash my face with a 9. Brush my teeth with an 8. Shower in 10s and rub 9 in my hair. Get out of the shower and rub 9 lotion all over my largest organ, a direct portal to my blood stream. Put 10 makeup all over my face, eyes, cheeks. Ride to work with an air freshener in my car rated 10. Clean my desk with 10 rated disinfectant wipes. Wrap up the day eating gluten and removing my makeup with a 10-rated product. Then sleep all night with the one thing my mom still questions as the reason she got cancer...

...plastic. Yes, for two straight years I slept with plastic marinating in my mouth. I had the popular Invisalign braces when I was 18-20 years old, and my lifelong retainers that I still wear today are made from plastic. This was definitely my 'Holy Shit' moment of figuring out how I arrived at an autoimmune diagnosis.

During my Invisalign treatment, every two weeks I had to visit the dentist to get re-fitted for new retainers. I was 18 and knew little-to-nothing about holistic health, but I always felt like this process was toxic for my body. Every two weeks I would sink my teeth into melted, purple plastic that reeked of chemicals so bad that I would get nauseous from the fumes while I sat there with my mouth wide open, lips cracking, waiting for this retainer fitting to dry. The dentist would then put on his purple latex gloves to tug and pull inside my mouth, trying with all his might to get this now hardened plastic retainer out. He then shipped it to the Invisalign company to have my new, bi-weekly retainer created. Did I mention he glued plastic 'clips' on my teeth so the retainers would lock in and not move?

For 18 months, I had freaking Gorilla Glue in my mouth.

The mouth, especially under the tongue, is a direct connection to the blood stream. This Invisalign procedure was literally no different than being hooked up to an IV of melted plastic for two years straight. The moment I realized this, is the moment my Hashimotos diagnosis did not surprise me at all.

———◆———

After coming to the conclusion that I needed a hazmat suit to enter my own bathroom, I ran to the kitchen to grab a trash bag to throw away all of my toxic bathroom products.

As I turned the corner to enter the kitchen I stopped to stare at the sink. Oh shit. I ripped out my iPhone from my back pocket and opened the app to scan my pretty pink dish soap. Rates a 10. My blue window cleaner: 8. I walk around the corner to the laundry room and grab my dryer sheets, loaded with fragrance. 10. I soon realize that any product that contains artificial fragrance automatically rates a 10... so my entire laundry room was bursting with cancer causing ingredients. All day, and all night, my body was wrapped up in chemicals. *This can't be real.*

———◆———

The afternoon sun was beginning to set as I walked down the stairs of our third floor apartment with an oversized trash bag in tow, full of bathroom supplies, makeup, and cleaning products. I felt wasteful throwing all of these products away, but I was done living in a chemical soup. If I was going to be my own best doctor, I knew what I had to do; it was time to eliminate ALL hormone disrupting chemicals from my home. I was going all or nothing. As I approached the big community dumpster, I swung the bag over my shoulder and tossed it in. As I turned around to walk into my new, toxic-free life, I stopped to lift my hands to my nose....

...the trash bags were scented with fragrance.

So where do you begin?

Step 1: Download the Think Dirty app. As of August 2017, it is compatible with both iPhone and Android. Get it on your phone and prepare to use it as much as Facebook. Another great online resource is the Environmental Working Group. (www.ewg.org)

Step 2: Begin scanning every product in your home. If they score high, click on the ingredients list to see why. Read about each ingredient and its health impact. I know, most of them have names you can't pronounce. But soon you'll be able to recognize which ingredients are bad when you're out shopping, whether you have your phone with you or not.

*Rule of Thumb: *Anything with 'fragrance' or 'parfum' will automatically rate a 10 and should be avoided at all costs. The word Fragrance is a blanket term for over 3,000 hidden chemicals. According to the Environmental Working Group, several of these chemicals are very harmful: 'Of the 3,163 chemicals listed [under the term fragrance], several stand out as particularly toxic: phthalates, octoxynols and nonoxynols. Phthalates are potent hormone disruptors linked to reproductive system birth defects in baby boys. Octoxynols and nonoxynols break down into persistent hormone disruptors, as well.' ~ EWG.org*

Step 3: Work towards using products that rate 3 or lower, and are always fragrance free — unless they are scented with essential oils.

Some Brands I love:

(All rate 3 or lower on Think Dirty)

Makeup: W3LL People, Gressa Skin, ZuZu Luxe.

Hair: Acure Organics and Avalon Organics.

It took me years to find organic hair care products that

were both affordable and didn't dry my hair out. These two brands hit the mark. I use Avalon Organics Lemon clarifying shampoo & Acure deep conditioner.

*Thyroid Hair Loss: *Doesn't it suck? Thinning hair was the first symptom I had that made me question if something was up with my hormones. As you regain balance of your hormones, your hair will naturally grow back. But to speed things up, use Castor Oil treatments! I rub the oil on my eyebrows and lashes every night and it has helped my hair grow back immensely. My eyebrows are actually fuller than they've ever been in my life! You can also rub it on the scalp, but it's a very thick oil so it may take a few washes to get it out. My favorite herbal supplements to support hair regrowth are Silica and Horsetail.*

Skin: I love Acure facial serums and moisturizers for Summer months.

Jojoba oil + Frankincense essential oil is my nightly ritual! Frankincense is *amazing* for wrinkles, brown spots and acne.

Dr.Bronner's is hands down the best soap on the market. It doubles as dish soap, laundry soap, and it's bio-degradable!

Derma-e is another clean brand. I love their makeup remover. *Never underestimate plain old coconut oil! Great for removing makeup but also for naturally moisturizing skin and hair.

Cleaning: I love Seventh Generation, but I mainly focus on anything that is fragrance and dye free. I've also started to make my own products at home with basic items like baking soda, vinegar, and essential oils.

Young Living Essential Oils

Do you believe in synchronicity? In 2016 I was living in Charleston, SC and, late one summer afternoon, a bad round of storms rolled through my little island town. If you know me, you know I love a good thunderstorm. So, I ran to the beach right after the storm passed to take a long walk and absorb the negative ions. I had the place to myself — just how I like it. But as I'm walking, I see the cutest little family off in the distance. It's a woman with her young daughter and an old yellow lab just chillin' in the sand. I think to myself: *'That will so be me when I have a child someday.'*

As I walk by them, I can't help but stop to say hello. I mean, we were the only ones on what appeared to be a deserted island, and these three had such a beautiful energy to them. As it turns out, this woman named Elyse was a chiropractor and very much into holistic health — much like myself, as I was halfway through my health coach program at IIN. We instantly bonded over our love for plants over pills and she introduced me to Young Living essential oils.

These oils played such a vital role in bringing my thyroid back into balance that I have no doubt in my mind that my meeting with Elyse was divinely planned.

Back in 2014, when I first ransacked my apartment and threw away all toxic products, I found in my research that essential oils can really assist the body in removing toxins and restoring hormonal harmony. Up until I discovered Young Living, I was using cheap essential oils that I purchased at department stores or Amazon. I would rub these oils on my neck every night and diffuse them in my apartment. I thought I was doing everything right, but I failed to realize that the essential oil bottle said 'not for internal use' — Red flag! Anything you put *on* your body should be able to go *in* your body.

I have since tossed those oils in the trash and stick with

Young Living only. Their farms are 100% organic, non-GMO and every single oil is safe to consume. How do they keep pests from ruining their crop? Spray a dilution of peppermint oil on them! *(I'll never forget when I learned that. You hear that America? Peppermint > Pesticides)* Not only that, but they have a blend called Endoflex that is specifically targeted towards thyroid balance. (The fact that it's product number is 3333 is just another sign.) It's a blend of Spearmint, Sage, Geranium, Myrtle, German Chamomile and Nutmeg. I call this blend my "Thyroid Medication" - I rub it on my neck and vitaflex points on my feet every morning and night.

Not only does Young Living provide my monthly 'thyroid meds' but I soon discovered that they are all about an entirely toxin-free life. They believe that the only way to gain full benefit from essential oils is if your entire life is toxin free. *Now you're talkin' my language.* This includes diet and lifestyle. If you are eating fast food every day but rubbing Endoflex on your neck at night, you are only gaining half the benefit. Your body will use the oils to detox the chemicals from the fast food instead of healing and repairing your thyroid. Get it?

Young Living offers cleaning products through their massively popular 'Thieves' line. Thieves is a highly anti-bacterial oil made from Clove, Lemon, Cinnamon Bark, Eucalyptus and Rosemary oils. It's called Thieves because there's an old story that dates back to when the plague was running rampant. A group of three men would rob the graves of the deceased but never catch the plague. When they were arrested, the law agreed to let them go if they shared their secret on how they were able to never get sick. The secret to their immortality: this blend of essential oils.

I'll never forget learning about Thieves at my first essential oils class. We took turns passing around a single slice of white bread in a plastic sandwich bag; half of it was covered in mold while the other half looked fresh out of the oven. As it was my turn to examine the bread, I looked up with a scrunched face at the woman presenting and asked:

"What in the world this is? Half Rotten bread?"

She explained that inside that bag was a slice of bread from over six month's ago. One half was sprayed with Thieves cleaning solution and the other half was not. This was just one example showcasing how powerful plant based cleaners are at killing bacteria. I was convinced! So now my home is filled with Thieves cleaning supplies and I'll never look back.

*To learn more about Endoflex, Thieves, and replacing every toxic product in your home with essential oils, visit my website www.evolve2health.com and enroll under my Health Coach practice! Bonus: You will be added to Facebook groups with endless resources to help you on your toxic-free lifestyle journey, including me as your personal guide.

**I just want to note for my own satisfaction: This is not a Multi-Level Marketing push. I was hesitant to sign up for Young Living due to my own negative viewpoint towards MLM's. When I finally removed that block, I was welcomed into a whole new world of healing. The vast majority of those who both use and distribute Young Living are some of the smartest, most health conscious families I've ever met. Come join us!

CHAPTER 3
Head & the Heart

"Are you speaking your truth?"

We've arrived. The final, and in my opinion, most important chapter of the book. I actually almost made the entire book on what I'm about to share with you…

On top of the physical pieces of the puzzle (diet and lifestyle) there is also a strong spiritual/emotional connection to a dysfunctional thyroid. You see, the thyroid gland lies right in the middle of a very busy, very important highway. This highway connects your head to your heart. When these two are at odds with each other, a bad "traffic jam" can occur.

As I've evolved into my personal style of health coaching, I've really started to centralize my focus on the importance of emotions to our physical health. If a client walks in with red eyes from crying the night before, kale is the last thing we are going to talk about. At the Institute for Integrative Nutrition, they taught us something very significant about nutrition. There are two ways to categorize it:

Primary Food refers to everything that feeds us that is not food. These are things such as our careers, relationships, spirituality, physical activity, finances, education, environment, social life, and other lifestyle factors that play an equal if not more significant role in the quality of our lives than what is on our plates.

Secondary Food is the actual food we eat: fruits, vegetables, grains, proteins, and fats. Secondary Food does not provide the fulfillment Primary Food provides, but, oftentimes we use it to suppress our hunger for Primary Food.

If our Primary Food is balanced and fulfilled, eating healthy secondary food will come naturally. It is when an area of our primary food becomes unbalanced that we tend to overeat or make poor decisions on what to put on our plate.

I started to notice that throughout my coaching sessions, once we started to dive deep into Primary Food, all of a sudden teaching my clients about vegan recipes and sharing the latest gluten free treats didn't matter. The center of our conversations revolved around why they would get so nauseous thinking about going back to work on Monday. Or why it's so uncomfortable to hug their family members even when they know they love them.

Let's use children as an example: Do you ever notice that kids are never really hungry? When they are outside playing, you have to yell for them multiple times to come inside and eat dinner. Why is that? Their Primary Food is full. It is a time in life for them that they have little to no responsibilities, and they (hopefully) feel very loved and cared for. Eating is not on the top of their priorities list, and doesn't fulfill them nearly as much as climbing a tree.

My favorite example to showcase the importance of Primary Food: **Love.** Oh, the honeymoon phase in a relationship! You know the feeling. You meet a new partner and fall head over heels for each other. Your blood pumps every time you see their name pop up on your phone. You feel more attractive, knowing there's someone out there who only has eyes for you. You feel wanted, knowing there's someone out there thinking about you all day. Every love song on the radio suddenly becomes about you two... and life is just perfect. Everything feels fulfilled and complete.

Do you ever notice that during times of such bliss, you aren't really hungry, or craving anything in particular? In fact, a lot of people lose weight when they first begin new relationships. A whole day can pass by without feeling a ping of hunger. You can go on a dinner date with your lover, order the cheesiest pizza, and be full on only one slice versus your usual three. Your Primary Food is overflowing!

Typically, when a piece of our 'Primary Food Pie' is imbalanced, be it career or relationships, it is because we haven't been living our truth. Our heart is communicating one thing, but our brain is telling us 'No.'

"I can't quit my job that stresses me out — I have bills to pay."

"I can't showcase my talent to the world — I'm not good enough."

When I began my thyroid healing journey and learned about the head and the heart connection, it began a completely new cycle of life for me that involved deep inner reflection and lots of releasing. I'm still going through this phase as I write this book. We all struggle at some point in our lives to speak up and say how we really feel. Unfortunately, I have been struggling with a repressed inner voice for the vast majority of my life.

My story:

I was born into a broken family. My brother, only 18 months older than me, had Aspberger's but nobody knew it. My mother and father were not in love, and my father was an abusive alcoholic who was never around. My mother suffered from her own childhood traumas and depression. I was born into a family where negativity was the norm, and showing emotion was a rarity. And speaking how you truly felt? Unheard of. From day one, I am taught to be uncomfortable giving someone a hug or saying the words 'I love you'.

As my brother and I grew up, his Aspberger's took center stage. His indifference to society caused for lots of trouble at school and intense outbursts at home. This both embarrassed me and made me so sad inside. I loved my big brother and thought he was so much fun, but the outside world didn't view him the same. This really took a toll on my mother too. Sadly, I had a front row seat to witness the pain and confusion that comes with being a single parent raising a child on the autism spectrum.

To fill in the role of a missing father, I inevitably fell into the role of a caregiver. I was six years old and keeping our apartment in the projects as clean as a whistle. I took care of pets, helped with dinner and dishes, and vacuumed the carpet every single day. I didn't mind either — the look of relief on my mom's face when she arrived home from her tiring job as a nurse was all the reassurance I needed to keep going. For a brief moment in time, I got to see a golden glimpse of her being happy, and that was all that mattered to me. I made sure I performed well at school and stayed out of trouble, always keeping my mouth shut. I never shared my troubles or worries with people, because I believed combining them with my brother's issues would be way too much for anyone. My heart was telling me to talk about my emotions, but my brain was telling me to keep quiet because we sure didn't need anything else on our plate.

Despite all of this, I still stayed true to my soul. When I wasn't cleaning toilets, I was outside climbing trees, catching frogs and always listening to music on my yellow Walkman. I loved nature, animals, and music more than anything in the world. I felt like I could be myself around them — troubles and all. When I climbed to the top of the tree to watch the sun set, it didn't matter if I had a dad or not. When I was riding my bike blasting music, the images of my mom in tears, getting a hug from her friend as they walked into a church basement to get free bread and milk for us, dissipated from my mind.

In the sixth grade, that all came to a crash when someone made fun of my friend for having hairy legs. As this girl laughed and gagged about the dark hair covering my friend's legs, I looked down at my own and noticed they were covered in layers of long blonde hair. Surely people would notice and begin to make fun of me too. That day when I got home from school, instead of strapping on my rollerblades, I filled up a bath tub and grabbed my mom's rusty razor as I asked her to teach me how to shave my legs. I was doing what society and my ego wanted me to do... and ignoring the call of my soul, that just wanted to grab the Walkman and go rollerblading.

Soon after that, soccer shorts turned into tight jeans and morning routines took a bit longer as I all of a sudden couldn't leave the house without makeup. I traded climbing trees for AOL Instant Messenger. I stopped listening to my Walkman and started listening to gossip from friends. Sure, this provided me with a temporary high, but the drama and bullying moved in like a hurricane as my soul went from a blazing sun to a flickering candle.

I began sacrificing my soul identity for the sake of attention. I just wanted people to notice me, and for boys to think I'm beautiful. I think this urge for affection stemmed from not getting attention at home and having no father figure in my life. It was such a gaping void, and filling it with friends and boys provided temporary relief. Sadly, my mother is not very good in relationships either. She has boyfriends come and go like the wind.

I didn't realize the emotional toll this took on me until my late 20s. It always felt like just as I was about to jump over that awkward line of calling them 'dad', they would disappear. I stepped out of my comfort zone to allow these new men into my life, live with them, eat with them, form sibling-like bonds with their children, only for them to be gone one day. Just like my biological father from my first five years of life. This pattern continues for years, and I never once spoke up about it. I was a professional at sweeping emotions under the rug, because that's the lifestyle I was born into. It was a coping mechanism. One thing I now know is, unreleased emotions will always manifest as physical dis-ease later in the body.

During high school, I'm severely bullied. Mostly by girls that were once my best friend, who I opened up to, allowed into my home and around my family. The bullying was usually due to insecure girls deflecting their jealousy onto me by giving me the name 'slut' or 'homewrecker'. I was even bullied by boys. I have yet to discern why I was bullied so much, perhaps it was because I never fought back due to my habit of keeping the peace.

As my bullies confronted me in hallways, followed my school bus to try and 'kick my ass' in front of my own home, or even when they paintballed my mother's house she worked so hard to purchase on her own, I never confronted them. I never told those lost souls how I really felt. Of course, I felt anger, and afraid, and sad. But I never released any of it. While being pushed into a locker, I kept a poker face. As I peeled off dried bologna from my first car I worked so hard to afford, I didn't say a word. When the guidance counselor at my high school told me I needed to have lunch in her office in order to protect me from bullies, I happily obliged instead of standing up for myself and how unfair that was. I was on a mission to never rock the boat. Never add any more worries to my mom's plate. Just like I learned to do when I was young, I swept it all under the rug... assuming the rage would just go away one day.

When I was 18 and finally graduated high school, I felt as though I was sitting in the middle of dust and debris after an emotional explosion. I had my first serious boyfriend, but I knew I didn't love him. I had barely any friends left, and no idea what I wanted to do with my future. With the little energy my soul had left, it began picking up the pieces and building a protective wall around me.

I defaulted to a local state college mostly because my boyfriend and friends went there, ignoring my inner voice that said *'pursue music or something in the arts'*. I still remember keeping the web page for Full Sail University open on my laptop for months, but my ego told me I wasn't good enough. At age 19, I finally broke up with my boyfriend, which was one of the very first times I ever spoke my truth. I broke his heart, but I spoke honestly about how I felt and, as he drove away, I'll never forget how weightless and free I felt.

The very next day I started a new diet/workout regimen and got down to the lowest weight I had ever been. I was no longer eating to cover emotions! I was dating for fun, excelling in my college classes, and even decided to move across the country to study the hospitality industry in Las Vegas. The following year was one of the best years of my life. I went from celebrating my 19th birthday in an empty Applebee's to celebrating my 20th birthday going on rides that dangle you over the Las Vegas strip with my new, wild, best friend. All of this because I spoke my truth! I met so many amazing people in Las Vegas who became lifelong friends… I finally found my tribe.

Later that year, I met my husband.

Oh Mitch. He's such an angel. They always tell you growing up that when you meet 'the one' you'll just know. Well, I never believed in that — given my upbringing — but when I first ran into Mitch's arms for a big hug on our first date… I felt home. I didn't feel butterflies, I didn't feel lust, I just felt like I finally arrived home. A place where I didn't have to hide anything or hold anything in.

As everything in my life feels unstable and uncertain, Mitch is the one constant. He has taught me what unconditional love looks like and showed me how comfortable hugs and 'I love you' can be. *He was actually one of my first friends when I was eight years old and just moved to New Hampshire from Indiana. I guess you could say we are elementary school sweethearts…but that's another book.*

When I was 22 years old, Mitch asked me to marry him. We had talked about getting married before, to the point where I would say I almost pushed it to unnaturally happen. I recall always saying that before we got our own place together, I wanted a rock on my finger. Looking back, I have no idea why. I was so lost and confused about life; I had so much growing up to do and didn't even know it. He asked me two days after my 22nd birthday, on Decem

ber 8th. I was very sick with the flu when Mitch pulled me off the couch to say he had one more birthday surprise for me. As he nervously led me to my childhood bedroom, we began an awkward game of 'hot or cold'…. I started to suspect this was it. I couldn't tell if the nausea was my flu or intuition revving up. As I walked closer to a conch shell on my desk, Mitch's face flushed as he said 'REALLY WARM!'. I picked up the shell and saw the black ring box. I was about to throw up and had no idea why. *This is what you've been pushing for, Steph.* I didn't want to turn around and look at him, because I knew what was next. But I robotically turned around and Mitch was on one knee with a really uncomfortable smile on his face, as he says,

"Will you marry me?"

I still don't know why I was so hesitant during his proposal. I think it's because emotionally charged moments are programmed into me to be extremely uncomfortable. Maybe it was years of social conditioning, of seeing guys come in and out of my life, that made me feel this way about committing my entire life to one person; I'm conditioned to believe it never works. My intuition nearly choked my throat so that I could not speak a word to answer him. Mitch remembers this. He always jokes to our friends and family that I almost said 'No' when he proposed because I silently stuttered before just nodding my head in a robotic 'Yes'.

It's not that I didn't love Mitch. That boy is something unworldly to me and has completely changed how I view love and life. He is the biggest blessing I have ever received. However, the following years would slowly reveal to me that the idea of marriage was something I never should've toyed with as a young 22-year-old who was still figuring out who she is and what life is all about. I hated picking out a wedding date and hated trying on dresses even more. I had nothing to do with designing the wedding invitations, because secretly I didn't care if they went out or not. I will never forget having a mental breakdown complete with silent sobbing as I found out my mom planned a surprise wedding shower for us. I didn't want to go to that! Or when Mitch's mother gifted me 'something blue' and as I looked at it with a very confused face, wondering why she would give me something blue, she explained the whole something borrowed, something blue tradition. *What the fuck is that? I don't want this, and I don't want to know.* I thought to myself. I could not understand why these awful, angry emotions boiled over during the wedding process; a time in life that is supposed to feel wonderful. This was so out of character for me.

One rainy afternoon a month after our wedding, Mitch drove me around town to hand in the paperwork that would officially change my last name. Again, intense emotions were buzzing through my body, almost uncontrollably. They would bounce from sadness to anger, but mostly anger. I felt like by giving up the name I was born with, I was handing over my identity to Mitch on a silver platter. Like here, take my world, tell me what to do and how to live my life til death do us part. *Ugh.* And I know what you're thinking, no one forced me to change my name, so why did I do it? Because something else inside my soul that I've swept under the rug my entire life was boiling to the surface; my anger towards my father. I wanted to get rid of his name and never be associated with his side of the family again. What made it worse was how frustrated I was that I had no idea what to do or which name to keep. I didn't want either of them, I didn't know what my truth was anymore...

...and six months later I was diagnosed with my Hashimotos Thyroid Disease.

———◆———

While my thyroid disease has been reversed and I have no active thyroid antibodies in my system, my TSH is still teetering on the edge of being hyperthyroid. I always say that I'm just one gluten-filled bagel away from being hyper again. So, why aren't they perfectly in the normal range? I know why, and the answer is this chapter. My head and heart are still having an internal battle while I try to come home to my truth, and my thyroid is ground zero for these mismatched energies.

At 27, just last year, I hit a breaking point. Call it a quarter life crisis, but I had a major breakdown because absolutely nothing in life felt right. I lived far away from all of my family. I was working a 9-5 job that had nothing to do with nature, music, or animals. I was drowning in student loan debt for a degree I never wanted, and I lived in a place I had no intention of planting roots.

How the hell did I stray this far away from my truth?

I developed panic attacks that kept me from driving for weeks at a time. I fell into waves of deep depression. It's ironic reflecting on this time, because a physical symptom I felt so strongly was dizziness. I'll never forget laying on the beach on Thanksgiving 2016. I was laying on a towel in the sand when I looked out into the horizon and saw the landscape flip upside down. It wouldn't stop. This spun me, literally, into a severe panic attack.

I was terrified to look up at the sky because it was always spinning or upside down. I feared that I would die and be stuck in this 'horrible life', in a suffocating black box, and never move on. I had to use all the willpower I had to remind myself that it wasn't real. This was my subconscious emotions manifesting into my reality. My soul had been upside down and all the gold coins of what I truly loved, who I truly was inside, were lost in a hurricane of lies.

You see, our neck bridges the head to the heart. In order to create hormonal harmony, these two must be delicately balanced. In energetic terms, we must be following our heart while also thinking logically with our head; it's a very delicate balance that definitely takes practice. When we are focused too much on logic, or following our heart without meditating on why, physical hormones can be affected. What butterfly shaped gland lies right in the neck, in the middle of this energy transfer? The thyroid. Also known as The Throat Chakra.

I was 26 when my mother-in-law Allison (one of those people I'm sure is my earth angel) planned a trip for me to see Cassadaga, Florida. This place is known as the psychic capitol of the world. Allison knew I was studying holistic health and had a passion for all things spiritual, so she was adamant that I visit this place. Of all the times I've been to Florida I had never heard of Cassadaga— it's a 'spiritual camp' full of psychic residents who devote their lives to the practice. It's been said that, in order to live within town limits, you must prove your intuitive abilities. On the front page of their website (www.cassadaga.org), you will find quotes like: 'As the sunflower turns it's face to the light of the sun, so Spiritualism turns the face of humanity to the light of truth.'

It was a warm January day when we were rolling down the highway in my jeep rental with directions to Cassadaga plugged into the GPS. We had just left an orange grove so, with a belly full of citrus, I was feeling so excited to mingle with like-minded people and see what this infamous town was all about. As soon as we got off the exit to make our way into this tiny town I began to feel the energy emanating from their grounds. Soon, the scenery changed from manicured palms to a rustic forest. When we drove past the Cassadaga welcome sign and started to see black cats roaming freely everywhere, I knew I was divinely guided here. This was no accident or coincidence. This was planned. I just knew that what I was about to experience was going to be a pivotal moment in my life…

We parked the jeep next to a rundown cottage with black cats crawling everywhere; on the porch, on top of the car, in the trees. It was quite the cliché sight. We walked by several shops with windows filled with crystals, sage, and tarot cards. Psychic readers perched at their tables watching your every move, hoping you would take a seat with them.

We made our way into the community center where they had a popular medium in town who was offering Chakra photos with her gigantic, state-of-the-art camera. As I watched people wait their turn to put on a black cape and step in front of the lens, I felt a pull to get mine done. I originally set out to speak with a psychic or have a tarot card reading done. Chakras interest me but I felt I knew enough about them already. But - I followed my internal compass and signed up to get my picture taken.

I grabbed a number and waited in line. I began sifting through photos on the table. Some people had bright, colorful auras while others had none. Some had chakras the size of a pencil mark while others had wide open chakras like the most vibrant pinwheels you've ever seen. *Yeah, that's what mine will look like…* so I thought.

They call my number and I step into the photo booth as a woman wraps a black cape around me as if I'm about to get a haircut. I put the palm of my hands on the arm rest that has sensors to help capture the energy in the chakras. Being a Sagittarius, I naturally make a goofy face and strike a pose. Everyone in the room laughs. I love it. I just knew my chakras would be blazing!

I step out of the booth and meet an old woman at the end of a long, school cafeteria sized table. She's the intuitive in charge of interpreting my photo. I sit down and start small talk with her while we wait for my photo to develop. Another woman walks over and slides it across the table to us. I tried to peek but she snatched it up quick. 'Ahhhh, a creative one I see!' she exclaims as she glances down at my photo. My aura in the photo is a bright red mixed with orange. I smile and say yeah, I just got into photography and really love it. I dream of working in the arts. 'Do you do it full time now?' she asked. 'No. Right now I work for a health insurance company.' I say with defeat.

She slides the photo over to me and my thoughts trail off as my focus is immediately drawn to my throat chakra. The tiniest faint blue circle is engulfed by an abundance of every other chakra. 'You aren't speaking or living your truth, my dear,' she calmly says. My ego flared with attitude, and in my thoughts, I snapped back, *UH...YES I AM!* While my heart softly whispered, *no, no you aren't.*

———————

As soon as I understood the importance of speaking your truth in order to heal the thyroid, it became clear to me why women suffer from thyroid imbalances much more than men. We are fresh out of a generation where women were second class citizens, unable to speak their truth. We still experience that form of sexism today.

When a man speaks up, he is a strong leader. When a woman speaks up, she is a moody bitch. For my male readers, you have it just as tough. Society has conditioned you to hold in your emotions. Crying is for wimps. If you show emotion, you are labeled as weak. These emotions will build up in your throat, your blue chakra, because your head has put up a wall against your heart. Our inner voices are stifled. Women are taught from infancy to be pretty, polite, and perfect. Men are taught to be strong, stand up for themselves, and never bow down.

Women are blessed with the gift of being creators of life. We grow babies in our wombs and naturally give up who we are to care for this precious new life. Our wants and desires inevitably take a back seat to our family's well-being. It is no wonder the vast majority of women are diagnosed with a thyroid disease in their late 20s - early 40s. This is the time we really give up who we are to become mothers! caregivers! We are putting on a mask at our career all day and sacrificing our wants and needs at night to make sure our family is content. Our head and our heart become completely unfamiliar to each other.

I believe that in order to fix this balance, we should practice feeling more comfortable sharing our truths. Are you working a job you truly love or do you just spend eight hours a day doing something mindless because it pays the bills? Do you really love your spouse or are you really preoccupied with creating a perfect life for Facebook? If you are not speaking your truth now, try digging deep — real deep — to figure out why. What are the things you did as a child that you no longer do now? Why not?

There is a book I love to refer to for clients when wondering what emotional event may have caused their physical disease. It's called 'Heal Your Body' by the late Louise Hay. (Ironically enough, as I type this, Louise passed away yesterday. May she rest in peace while we continue sharing her legacy.) When I flip through the index and get to Thyroid it says:

Probable Cause : Humiliation. *"I never get to do what I want to do. When is it going to be my turn?"*

Healing Affirmation: *"I move beyond old limitations and now allow myself to express freely and creatively."*

Hypothyroid:

Probable Cause: *Giving up. Feeling hopelessly stifled.*

Healing Affirmation: *"I create a new life with new rules that totally support me."*

Hyperthyroid:

Probable Cause: *Rage at being left out.*

Healing Affirmation: *"I am at the center of life and I approve of myself and all that I see."*

———◆———

So how do you begin speaking your truth?

Well, it's not easy. Speaking your truth is difficult — really difficult. You will lose friends, upset family members, and confuse others. Prepare for a lot of shocked faces. And you most certainly will not be able to fully heal this piece of the puzzle overnight. It is something you need to work at and practice every day. You're going to have days you're honest, and days you're not. Take a mental note of when you're not speaking your truth, and think about how you'll do it next time.

With so many resources at our fingertips today, I've found outlets for speaking my truth through social media. Remember in the beginning of the book, I told you how I conceived the idea for this book by taking hikes in the woods alone? That is the very first step I took to begin speaking my truth.

Sometimes, I would talk to myself in my head, other times out loud for the trees. No one got to hear my truth but the birds and the bugs. I would always head home from these hikes feeling 50lbs lighter in my heart and in my mind. After about a year of daily therapeutic walks, I decided to step it up and be even more vulnerable with my truth, so I started a blog. I had been reading a few popular blogs for years and always looked forward to the posts about real life. So, I started my own and called it Free Spirit Fun. I named it this because that was my truth - I was a free spirit, and all I want to do is make life fun. So, I blogged about my passion for travel and adventures.

What started out as a lighthearted blog, slowly morphed into deep posts about pain and struggles and trying to figure out life as a 20-something. I once wrote a post about the night my brother had his first grand mal seizure and I was the only one there to help him. I wrote that long post through shaking hands and had sweat dripping down my chest as I hit "Post". I'll never forget hitting enter, then slamming my laptop shut and anxiously pacing around the house.

Why the hell would you let people into your life, your home, and share such an intimately sad moment with the world, Steph?? I kept asking myself.

But, I figured I had nothing to lose. That was the first time I ever revealed my truth and became vulnerable on the internet for anyone to see. To my surprise, I woke up the following day to an inbox full of people admiring how brave I was, or old friends saying they had no idea I've been through such a traumatic event.

This inspired my most popular blog post to date, "20 Things I Learned in my Early 20s" — An article I wrote about all the things life has taught me in my 20s so far. I thought it was a very personal article, and wasnt sure if anyone would relate. But shortly after I posted it, my inbox filled up with people reaching out to share how much this post helped them and how they, too, have experienced similar life lessons.

I eventually stopped blogging to focus on my budding career as a health coach and, instead, focused my attention on instagram to continue sharing my truth. This little photo sharing app has led me to so many cherished friendships with sweet souls everywhere, from the plains of Oklahoma to the city of Singapore. These virtual friends have really helped me through hard times and helped me not feel so alone in my fear and anxiety. They have cheered me on and watched me evolve into the person I am today, and I can't believe a little app on my phone has provided me with such a blessing.

I can say without a doubt, that letting your guard down on social media and being real and authentic will lead to some of the most amazing connections and profound inner healing you couldn't even dream possible.

So, start writing! Text your thoughts on the notepad app in your phone. Handwrite them on paper. Start a blog. Write them on Instagram. Who cares if your audience is a single set of eyes or a thousand. Just by writing down your truth, you are releasing the emotional block in your throat chakra, clearing the way for the head and the heart to live in harmony once again. And when you close the final page of this book, and these words are long gone from your memory, I hope that you will always remember how absolutely important it is to live your truth. I love the quote that says,

> *"The planet does not need more successful people. The planet desperately needs more peacemakers, healers, restorers, story-tellers, and lovers of all kind."*
>
> —*Dalai Lama*

The earth desperately needs you to be you. Not what society tells you that you should be. Take care of yourself and never lose who you are for the sake of career or family. For the sake of fitting into society. Release emotions when you feel them, instead of sweeping them under the rug, hoping they will just go away. It's essential that you face the repressed emotions. *And hey, tears are just pent up emotions manifested as drops of water being released from your soul.* Cry it out. Let it all go. Turn your daydreams into your reality, and watch how full your Primary Food becomes. How with ease, everything in life, both physical and mental, just falls into place...

Conclusion

I'm not smart enough. I don't have a literature degree. No one will publish a book I write, and why would anyone buy it? These are the things I kept telling myself to delay writing this book and getting it out there. My own lack of self-confidence was preventing others out in the world from healing. I was hiding my truth from the world and, in turn, not helping the state of chaos that we are currently in. But, a famous quote that I live by, 'Your dreams are on the other side of fear' constantly reminds me to keep going. I don't care if my grammar is imperfect or I don't hold a Medical Degree. I have been in your shoes, felt all the symptoms, and sat on the same crinkly paper as the doctor walked in and handed me the same diagnosis. I genuinely care about you, and want you to live a vibrant life with an abundance of health. In the pharmacy world, a patient cured is a customer lost. In my world, a patient cured is a happier world for my future babies and grandbabies.

Read these words then read them again:

Your dreams are on the other side of fear.

To hold the hard copy of this book, full of research I battled through an autoimmune disease to learn, and how mentally hard I worked to push fear and vulnerability aside, I have to take a sincere moment to say, Thank you. Thank you for believing in me and purchasing my very first book.

This is a surreal moment for me, a girl who thought her life was going to be spent in a cubicle, not creating anything or helping the world heal. But, here I am, sitting in my new apartment in Denver, Colorado, about to submit this writing into a publishing service to bring this book to you. I have never felt happier, healthier, and more optimistic about my future in my life. *This can be you.*

Thyroid First Aid Kit is just scratching the surface of my writing career— I have a plethora of ideas in my mind that I would love to share with the world; with you. I have plans to begin a podcast show called *Lightworkers Lounge* to share even more of my healing stories with you in a more intimate way.

Find me at www.evolve2health.com or on Instagram @evolve2health to stay updated on new book releases and upcoming events.

I send you all of the love and light you need to begin your healing journey. Remember, I'm right there next to you. I've done everything you're about to do. When you're standing in the bread aisle at the grocery store overwhelmed with all of the gluten-free choices. When you're standing in Target scanning every bottle of shampoo with your Think Dirty App. Or when your palms are sweaty because you're about to tell someone how you truly feel… I'm right there with you.

Summary of the Thyroid First Aid Kit

"If a flower doesn't bloom, we don't just cut it out or uproot it. We fix the environment in which it grows. We change the soil, increase nutrients, add more light, more water. This is how Holistic Health approaches the human body..."

—*Alexander den Heijer*

Do not remove your thyroid or put a band-aid on it. First, fix the environment in which it grows.

1. **Remove Gluten.** It's not wheat that you're allergic to, it's the way we grow it. Heal your leaky gut!

   ***Always ask your healthcare practitioner to test for Thyroid Antibodies when you get your labs drawn.

2. **Replace toxic bath/beauty/cleaning products** with all natural ones ASAP. The most common beauty and household products are filled with endocrine disruptors, which could very well be why so many women are diagnosed with thyroid issues. Switch to all natural products and use the Think Dirty App to be sure a product is clean. Essential Oils are an excellent alternative.

3. **Speak your Truth.** Do not be afraid to say how you truly feel or put your desires first. Do not sweep emotions under the rug. Keep the highway between the head and the heart flowing freely...

Hire Stephanie Powers
to Speak at Your Next Event!

Stephanie has been speaking to groups and organizations about the thyroid and spiritual awakenings for the past 3 years. She's an expert on the endocrine system, mental health, and has helped countless clients achieve hormonal harmony through physical and emotional healing.

Author of Thyroid First Aid Kit and several on-line publications, Stephanie believes healing begins in the mind and only then will the physical body begin to follow suite. She believes the thyroid epidemic is something that needs more media attention, and that people need to stop accepting genetics as the reason for their disease.

When she's not speaking about the thyroid, she is teaching groups about the healing powers of essential oils and CBD oil.

For more information or to hire Stephanie for your next event, email evolve2health@yahoo.com or visit www.evolve2health.com

CITATIONS

1. Hay, Louise L. Heal Your Body: the Mental Causes for Physical Illness and the Metaphysical Way to Overcome Them. Hay House, 2012.

2. Rasa, Sharon L. Heal Hashimoto's: Start with the Gut. CreateSpace Independent Publishing Platform, 2016.

3. Axe, Dr. Josh. "4 Steps to Heal Leaky Gut and Autoimmune Disease - Dr Axe." Dr. Axe, 12 Sept. 2017, draxe.com/4-steps-to-heal-leaky-gut-and-autoimmune-disease/.

4. Frack, Lisa, and Becky Sutton. "3,163 Ingredients Hide behind the Word 'Fragrance.'" EWG, EWG, 2 Feb. 2010, www.ewg.org/enviroblog/2010/02/3163-ingredients-hide-behind-word-fragrance#.WYGvRq2ZP-Y.

5. "Genes Load The Gun — Lifestyle Pulls The Trigger." - Caldwell Esselstyn

6. "Primary Food vs Secondary Food" - Joshua Rosenthal, Institute for Integrative Nutrition.

7. "If a flower doesn't bloom, we don't just cut it out or uproot it. We fix the environment in which it grows. We change the soil, increase nutrients, add more light, more water. This is how Holistic Health approaches the human body…" - Alexander den Heijer

Made in the USA
San Bernardino, CA
25 November 2018